KETOGENIC DIET FOR BEGINNERS
HOW TO USE A KETOGENIC DIET FOR WEIGHT LOSS

KATYA JOHANSSON

Table Of Contents

Introduction

A ketogenic diet or as it is also called a keto diet, low carb, high fat diet, a diet low in carbohydrates. In this kind of diet the body produces ketones in the liver which are used as energy.

Ketones are a byproduct of rapidly burned fat. When ketones come out in the body above the normal level it means that ketosis is taking place in the body.

This means that the body has begun to utilize fat stores in the body as an energy source for its everyday functions.

The ketogenic diet is used by many people around the world because of its efficacy and knowledge about this diet and following exactly the rules, can help lose weight without compromising the overall health.

Ketosis is the metabolic state achieved through a ketogenic diet. The ketogenic diet trends to mimic the effects of fasting by reducing carbohydrate intake and by calorie restriction. By fasting, the body utilizes body fat instead of carbohydrates as the principal source of energy.

Most people consume high quantities of carbohydrates on a daily basis. When you eat carbs, your body will produce glucose and release insulin.

Our bodies are used to the routine of breaking these carbohydrates down and using them for energy production. Eating less than 15g carbohydrates per day will cause the body enter the state of ketosis. The lower we keep our glucose levels, the better the results will be.

A ketogenic diet should vary around 75 percent fat, 20 percent protein and 5 percent carbohydrates.

Usually ketosis is a result of reduced calorie and carbohydrate intake, but can also take place during periods of fasting such as during overnight sleep when the body's metabolism naturally enters the process of ketosis.

Especially beginners should have a complete overview of the diet to help them make an informed decision about the diet. As always, those with health problems should consult their medical health provider so that he can help them to adjust to the meal plan or to monitor them to ensure that the ketogenic therapy will not affect their health.

Chapter 1: How does the ketogenic diet work

When the body begins to enter a ketogenic state, it will use the glycogen which is a derivate of glucose, a form of energy storage in the liver and muscles.

In the first period of the keto diet there will likely be a decrease in energy, strength and endurance but, once the body adapted being in ketosis and using fat for energy, strength should return to normal. The body usually adjusts, but building muscle will be much more difficult without carbohydrates. Difficult, but possible. You have just to keep your protein intake high and eat a little surplus of calories.

There have been studies showing both favorable and adverse effects. The major health problem is eating a high amount of carbohydrates together with high amounts of fats. Limiting carbs with the keto diet will not result in the negative effects (as a result of high carbohydrate consumption). Excess carbs are will be stored as fat, so eating a high amount of carbohydrates can lead to fat gain and obesity, as well as lower activity levels, if not kept in check. But, again these issues tend to occur when you consume high amount of carbs and high amounts of fats, not just high amounts of fats like in the keto diet.

Our bodies contain a very few amount of enzymes for dealing with fats, which means, storing them for energy. When our bodies are facing a lack of glycogen, a lower consumption of carbohydrates and an increase in fat intake, they adjust by building up a new amount of these enzymes.

If there isn't a history of kidney disease or predisposition to kidney weakness or failure it is less likely to have problems. However, you should always check with a physician prior to starting a keto diet.

What should we know as beginners?

You should only follow this diet for a three to six month I order to reach the desired goal and because your body does need carbohydrates in the long term in order to maintain a very best function .A complete depletion of glycogen can lead to a lack of energy, a lethargic feeling, dizziness, headaches, and sometimes even flu-like symptoms.

During the diet period it's preferable to make the water and sodium intakes higher than normal in order to avoid to extension of those symptoms and make sure you get all the macros your body needs. Macronutrients (Macros) are the daily intake of fats, protein, and carbohydrates. You should keep your net carbohydrates at between 20 and 40 grams, but below 30 grams would be optimal, as the lower you can keep your amount of net carbs, the better the diet will work. A net carb is the amount of carbs you eat minus the fiber content.

During the time you will limit your carbohydrates intake, these carbs will be obtained from vegetables, nuts, and some dairy products.

A recommendable macronutrients intake:

- 65-75% fats,
- 20-30% protein,
- 5% or less of carbohydrates.

For this purpose, you have to avoid bread, pasta, potatoes, fried items, cereals, beans, legumes, fruit, and of course sweets.

Most of the desired macronutrients should come from meats (beef, chicken, fish, pork, bison, seafood, veal, eggs, etc.), green and leafy vegetables, and healthy fats/oils (olive, coconut, macadamia, grass-fed butter, etc.).

As snacks, a few things to keep on hand would be nuts and not sweetened nut butters (almond, cashew, sunflower, etc.), cheeses, and protein shakes.

Drink Liquids, Especially Water. Be sure to consume plenty of water. You need to replace the fluids you lose every day in different ways. This may help prevent constipation and dehydration. Other options are unsweetened tea, milk, and 100 percent fruit juice.

Chapter 2: Carb Intake Effects On Wakefulness And Sleeping Patterns

More than 50 million Americans don't get enough sleep. Yet good health is tied to a good sleep. There are countless benefits of good night sleep:

- The brain remains sharp

- The immune system is kept strong

- The waistline trim

- The skin looking youthful

- Lowers the risk of high blood pressure and heart disease.

Food deficiency has to be avoided, because many nutrient deficiencies (such as those of magnesium, zinc, tocopherols, retinol, EPA/DHA, choline, iodine, and B vitamins) seem to increase the risk of sleeping disorder or poor sleep quality. Eating a selection of high density foods helps in most cases.

Proper food timing helps with regulation of wakefulness and sleeping pattern. It is highly recommended to eat when you want to be awake. If you are starting a schedule, you should eat within 30 minutes of waking, to increase the waking/hunger response after sleep.

Gastric juices will start to be produced at that time of day, which increases wakefulness.

In order to achieve a good night sleep you should not eat within 2-3h of this sleeping time for optimal sleep quality.

The liver has a signal system that will mention to the body that it is time to be awake when it detects up to a certain amount of glucose. Carbohydrates should be consumed in the morning or in the middle of the day until there is still daylight.

To optimizing your diet for better sleep, you should eat a low carbohydrate, high fat diet, which will include lots of digestible fiber and lots of fast digesting foods including row food.

10 Foods that help to sleep well:

☐   Fish – (especially salmon, halibut and tuna) full of vitamin B6, which is needed to make melatonin a sleep-inducing hormone triggered by darkness.

☐   Yogurt - Dairy products like yogurt and milk contain significant doses of calcium—and recent research suggests that being calcium-deficient may make it difficult to fall asleep.

☐   Kale - Green leafy vegetables, such as kale and collards, also boast healthy doses of calcium. And research suggests that being calcium deficient may make it difficult to fall asleep.

☐   Almonds - are rich in magnesium, a mineral needed for quality sleep (and also helps cure headache). A study published in the Journal of Orthomolecular Medicine found that when the body's magnesium levels are too low, it makes it harder to stay asleep.

☐   Walnuts - Walnuts are a good source of tryptophan, a sleep-enhancing amino acid that helps make serotonin and melatonin, the "sleep" hormone that sets your sleep-wake clock. Additionally, University of Texas researchers found that walnuts contain own melatonin, which may help you fall asleep.

☐ Cheese – Grandma's tales tells that warm milk can make us sleepy, but the truth is any dairy product can do it. Calcium (found in cheese, yogurt, milk,) helps the brain use the tryptophan found in dairy to produce melatonin. Additionally, calcium helps regulate muscle movements.

☐ Tuna - Fish such as tuna, halibut, and salmon are high in vitamin B6, which are needed make melatonin and serotonin. Other foods high in B6 include raw garlic.

☐ Pistachio nuts – have also a high content of B6.

☐ Shrimp and Lobster - Another good source of tryptophan, crustaceans like shrimp or lobster may help to sleep.

☐ Elk - This meat has tryptophan (carbohydrates in very little amount help the tryptophan reach the brain).

Chapter 3: Food Nutrient Density

Nutrient density means, how many nutrients you get from a food, compared with the number of calories it contains. In other words nutrient dense foods give us the most nutrients for the fewest amounts of calories. It gives us a very concentrated amount of valuable nutrients especially in whole, organically-grown foods. This organically grown foods are the healthiest foods.

These aims are obtained in the best way by foods with optimal nutrient density, and nutrient density is the best way for a healthy diet.

As reported by Medical Daily:

'Shifting the focus away from calories and emphasizing a dietary pattern that focuses on food quality rather than quantity will help to rapidly reduce obesity, related diseases, and cardiovascular risk,' the research team said in a statement"

Examples of high nutrient density foods:

☐   Hearts, brains and liver. Protein helps build and maintain muscle and skin, and it is advisable to include protein in our daily diet.

☐   Fish, shellfish, seaweed. These foods tend to be low in saturated fats.

☐   Green leafy, cruciferous, mushrooms. Vegetables, fruits, grains and beans give our body phytochemicals. Phytochemicals are natural compounds such as beta-carotene lutein (improve sight), and lycopene (fights cancer).

☐   Sunflower, pumpkin, chia are rich in good fat.

☐   Bone broth. Bones have lots of protein and collagen, the protein matrix in bones

☐   Egg yolks the high good cholesterol HDL contents of the eggs stimulates the serotonin receptors.

☐   Dairy products should be among the foods we choose every day. These products provide calcium and vitamin D and they also provide protein and potassium.

Chapter 4: The Benefits Of The Ketogenic Diet

In this regard the type of fat consumed is of crucial importance. The most recommended fat is the MCFA-s group (medium-chain fatty acids) like coconut oil, since this is the easiest type of fat for the body to burn as fuel. Therefore coconut oil is the most AND highly recommended. Another option to obtain short-chain fatty acids is from raw dairy products and other sources of fat from nuts especially sprouted nuts, seeds especially chia seeds, avocado, non-starchy vegetables, and organic meats.

The benefits of the ketogenic diet:

☐ Improved cholesterol due to improved triglyceride and cholesterol levels from arterial buildup

☐ Improved focus and energy as insulin spikes and crashes are minimized due to decrease in carbohydrate consumption

☐ Improved blood sugar since insulin levels are kept lower

☐ Increase in weight loss as the body is burning fat as its primary fuel source, and limiting carbohydrates tends to decrease overall caloric intake

☐ Decrease in hunger due to satiety provided by fats and proteins as well as increased vegetable intake

☐ Aids Weight Loss

☐ Aids in cases of Alzheimer's

☐ Is a natural treatment for dementia

☐ Helps rarefy the amount of epilepsy seizures

☐ Helps fighting cancer

The weight loss following a ketogenic condition is due to the fact that this diet increases our body's capability to use fat as its principal energy source and therefore reduces the body's fat stores, including the visceral fat which is the fat pile around the midriff. They can diminish appetite.

Reducing carbohydrates from the diet ensures that no accumulation of calories is stored in the body cells. The ketogenic diet works by eliminating carbohydrates from the diet and keeping the body's carbohydrate stores almost empty, preventing too much insulin from being released during meals. With less insulin around, the body starts burning its own body fat, helping you lose weight quickly. Moreover, the body will continue to burn fat even while we're sleeping. That means the body is burning fat every night.

The ketogenic diet is a high fat diet, it will not raise our cholesterol or increase our risk for heart disease. Heart disease is caused by inflammation, influenced mostly by the intake of trans fats and sugar, not by heart-healthy fats. So if we want to lose weight, reduce our risk of cancer, and improve our blood sugar, a ketogenic diet may be the right diet for you.

The ketogenic diet aids in cases of type 2 diabetes especially for those with type 2 diabetes who are not on insulin. (Diabetics on insulin should contact their medical provider prior to starting a ketogenic diet as insulin dosages may need to be adjusted.)

Coconut ketogenic diet:

Evidence shows that a ketogenic diet is a natural treatment for dementia, able to cure its symptoms completely and support the brain nerve system. We know that a diet made up of around 70 percent healthy fat helps the brain function much better.

When we start a keto diet, we'll want to make sure our plan ahead of time. We want to know not only which foods to consume but also how to prepare them. We have to set a "diet" in general, therefore let me give you a notion of how to cook ketogenic tasty dishes.

Chapter 5: Breakfast Recipes

For breakfast, the best choice is vegetables, scrambled eggs with cheese and onions, mushrooms and spinach cooked in a lot olive oil and cheddar cheese, or 2 eggs served with sausages and bacon, along some salad.

Smoked salmon with avocado and cream cheese. All this ideas can make a delicious ketogenic breakfast.

Ketogenic coffee

Ingredients

- ☐ organic, mold-free coffee
- ☐ 2 tablespoons of coconut oil
- ☐ 2 tsp. of pastured butter
- ☐ Boiling water

Directions

1. Pour boiling water on the organic, mold-free coffee.
2. STIR in the coconut oil and 2 tsp. of pastured butter in it.
3. SERVE HOT.

ketogenic hot chocolate

Ingredients

☐   Organic row cacao
☐   Organic coconut fat milk
☐   2 tsp. of pastured butter

Directions

1.   Pour boiling water on the organic raw cacao.
2.   Stir in the coconut milk and the butter.
3.   Serve hot

Keto Frittata

Ingredients

- [ ] 12 large Eggs
- [ ] 9oz. bag Frozen Spinach
- [ ] 1 oz. Pepperoni
- [ ] 5 oz. Mozzarella Cheese
- [ ] 1 tsp. Minced Garlic
- [ ] 1/2 cup Fresh Ricotta Cheese
- [ ] 1/2 cup Parmesan Cheese
- [ ] 4 tbsp. Olive Oil
- [ ] 1/4 tsp. Nutmeg
- [ ] Salt and Pepper to Taste

Directions

1. Microwave frozen spinach for about 3-4 minutes, or until defrosted (but not hot).
2. Squeeze the spinach with the hands and drain of as much water as you can. Set aside.
3. Pre-heat oven to 375 F. Mix together all of the eggs, olive oil, and spices.
4. Whisk well until everything is combined.
5. Add in the ricotta cheese, parmesan cheese, and spinach. When adding the spinach, break it apart into small pieces.
6. Pour the mixture into a cast iron skillet, and then sprinkle mozzarella cheese over the top.

Cheese - Bacon Egg Clouds

Ingredients

- [ ] 2 eggs
- [ ] 3 slices of bacon
- [ ] A sprinkle of grated parmesan cheese
- [ ] A sprinkle of shredded cheddar cheese
- [ ] Salt and pepper

Directions

1. Preheat oven to 400F.
2. Fry up 3 slices of bacon in a pan. When finished, set aside and cut into small bite-size pieces.
3. Crack 2 eggs into a mixing bowl.
4. Separate the yolks and place them into a separate small bowl. Using a whisk or electric mixer, whisk the egg whites until they become fluffy and firm. The consistency should resemble whipped.
5. Spray a small baking or casserole dish with non-stick spray oil. When the egg whites are whisked and fluffy, spoon them on to the baking dish as one pile to form the "egg cloud".
6. Using a spoon, form two small holes in the egg cloud. Place your two egg yolks into the holes being very careful not to break the yolks!
7. Stick your bite-sized bacon pieces into the cloud wherever they will fit.

8. Sprinkle your desired amount of parmesan and cheddar cheeses over the cloud.

9. Sprinkle the cloud with dashes of salt and pepper.

Low Carb Sandwich

Ingredients

6 Keto cream cheese pancakes (double my recipe here)

4 slices of Turkey (I used maple cured)

4 slices Ham (I used rosemary ham)

2 cups shredded Swiss Cheese

Sugar free syrup

Directions

1. Once the pancakes are ready, separate the turkey and ham into four piles with two slices each. Two piles of turkey with two slices, and two piles of ham with two slices.

2. Add 1/2 cup of Swiss cheese to each pile.

3. Cook on medium-low (you can do it in the same pan that you cooked the pancakes), add a little more coconut oil, and cover with a lid until the cheese is melted. Then, just stack them up.

4. Add your bottom pancake, then a stack of turkey and cheese.

5. Then, another pancake and a stack of ham on top.

6. Finally, another pancake and a little cheese on top.

7. Add it back to the frying pan on low heat, with a lid.

8. Drizzle the low-carb / sugar-free syrup over the top, just add a little bowl of syrup so you can dip it instead.

Bacon Keto Pancakes

Ingredients

1 Cup Carbquik

1 Egg

½ Cup Heavy Cream•¼ Cup Water

½ Cup Unsalted Butter, Melted

1 Tbsp. Sugar Free Vanilla Syrup

½ Tsp Baking Soda

8 Slices Bacon

Directions

1. Cook bacon either in the oven or on the stove.
2. Melt butter in the microwave.
3. Mix together the Carbquik and the baking soda.
4. Add the liquid ingredients and mix.
5. Heat pan over medium-high heat and then spray with Pam.
6. Spoon a glob of batter onto the pan, try not to make them too big or else they won't flip, add bacon.
7. When bubbles start forming near the center, or the edges start to brown, flip.
8. Cook for an additional minute.

Microwave Flax Muffins

Ingredients

1 egg

1 splash of heavy whipping cream

1 to 2 tsp. sweetener of your choice

1 pinch salt

1 tsp. vanilla extract

4 tbsp. ground flax meal

unsweetened cocoa powder

Directions

1. Mix in a microwave save bowl and microwave for 1 to 1 and a half minutes.
2. If it gets too dry, pitch a little piece of butter on top of the finished muffin and let it melt in.
3. Add 1 tbsp. or so of unsweetened cocoa powder.

Chapter 6: Lunch – Main Dishes Recipes

One of the best choices to have for lunch is a salad made from non-starchy vegetables. I recommend avoiding grains, starchy vegetables, sugar, sweet fruits, milk and yogurt and if at all, no more than 15 gr. of carbohydrates.

Good choices are leafy greens, such as arugula, lettuce and radicchio, cucumbers, avocado and cherry tomatoes, canned tuna, chicken breast, beef, boiled eggs, cheese, bacon, almonds, walnuts or macadamia nuts, and a low-carb salad dressing.

Christmas Turkey

Ingredients

2 thin cut rashers of streaky bacon

100g raw turkey breast escallops - 1 or 2

15g (4 -5) walnut halves, roughly chopped

15g (8-10) fresh or frozen cranberries, thawed if frozen

Pinch of dried thyme

Black pepper

60 gr. tender stem broccoli

60 gr. Brussels sprouts, trimmed

Directions

1. Preheat an oven to 190°C, (fan oven 170°C).

2. The turkey needs to be rolled up, so a thin cut is ideal. You may need to flatten a thick escalope by placing between cling film and tenderizing (pounding) briefly with a rolling pin

3. Cut a square of foil and place on a clean surface. Put the bacon rashers side by side in the middle of the foil and place the turkey escalope on top.

4. In a small bowl mix together the walnuts, cranberries and herbs and season with black pepper.

5. Spoon this onto the middle of the escalope.

6. Roll up the turkey with the bacon to make a parcel.

7. Crunch together the sides and top of the foil and place on a baking sheet.

8. Cook for 20 minutes, then open the top carefully so not to lose the cooking juices.

9. Return to the oven for 10 minutes to allow the bacon to brown a little.

10. Meanwhile steam the Brussels sprouts and broccoli.

11. Serve the turkey and its cooking juices with the green vegetables.

Smoked Cod With Stir Fried Vegetables

Ingredients

150g undyed smoked cod or haddock, preferably sustainably sourced.

1 small leek or 100g leek, cut into 1cm slices

1 head (about 100g) pak choi (bok choy), roughly sliced

1 tsp vegetable oil

1-2 tbsp. water

2 garlic cloves

Directions

1. Preheat the oven to 190°C (fan oven 170°) or gas mark 5.
2. Pour 4 tbsp. water into a small ovenproof dish and add the fish.
3. Add garlic.
4. Bake for 15-20 minutes until the fish flakes easily.
5. Meanwhile heat the oil in a non stick pan or wok, and add the leek and bock choy.
6. Stir fry over a high heat, adding the water to prevent sticking.
7. When the vegetables are just wilted serve on a warmed serving plate, and top with the fish.
8. Serve immediately.

Keto Burger

Ingredients

Cream of Tartar

6 Eggs

180g Cream Cheese

1kg Beef

Lettuce

Garlic

Herbs Straight up,

Sauces

1kg of beef mince

Directions

1. Separate egg whites from the yolks.
2. Mix 1/4 teaspoon, of cream of tartar, and using an electric beater, mix them for at least five minutes in a small container to make them whip up properly.
3. Mix the six yolks, and 180g of cream cheese, beating until 90% of the lumps are gone from the mixture.
4. When you have both a bowl of whites, and mixed yolk and cream cheese, combine them, and fold them into one another, preserving as much of the air that you can
5. To make them into buns, use a spring form pan, line the bottom, side optional, with baking paper, and pour in the mixture.

6. Pour half the mixture in at a time, and bake this at 150°C for at least 20 minutes, or until it browns slightly. This is how it looks when it's done.

7. Mix beef with two cloves of garlic, some olive oil, and mixed herbs. Knead the additions through in a big bowl.

8. When you're done, load this into the spring form pan, flattening it out into an even surface in a 9″ pan.

9. Put it in the oven at 180°C until done.

10. You should take it out to drain the fluids from time to time.

11. Now you have two buns, and a patty.

12. Take one patty and put down a layer and place the meat patty on top of cheese.

13. Then a layer of cheese on top.

14. Add some lettuce, then the top bun.

Crockpot Buffalo Chicken

Ingredients

6 Frozen Chicken Breasts

1 Bottle Frank's Red Hot sauce

½ Packet Hidden Valley Ranch

3 tbsp. butter

Directions

1. Put the chicken in the crockpot.
2. Pour the hot sauce over chicken and sprinkle ranch over top.
3. Cover and cook on low for 6 hours.
4. Shred, add butter, and cook on low heat for 1 hour uncovered.

Kalua Pork

Ingredients

1 4-6 lb pork shoulder

1 Tbsp. liquid smoke, Hickory

2-3 tsp. sea salt (depends on the meats size)

Directions

1. Wash and pat dry the pork roast and place in the slow cooker.
2. Pierce all over with a fork, pour the liquid smoke evenly over the roast and sprinkle with the sea salt.
3. Place the lid of the slow cooker on and set the time for 8-12 hours on low heat.
4. Check at about 8 hours if it's enough cooked .
5. If not done let go 4 hours more, checking every hour.
6. Either remove the pork from the pot and shred with a fork and return to pot or shred in the pot when it's done.
7. You can remove some of the liquid and shred
8. Add some back in the slow cooker, to keep the pork from drying out

Lasagne Meatballs

Ingredients for the meatballs

- [ ] 1 lb sweet or hot Italian sausage
- [ ] 1 lb ground chuck (or turkey if you prefer)
- [ ] ⅓ cup almond flour
- [ ] 2 eggs
- [ ] 1 Tbsp dried parsley
- [ ] 1 tsp kosher salt
- [ ] ¼ tsp red pepper flakes
- [ ] ½ tsp garlic powder
- [ ] ½ tsp onion powder
- [ ] ¼ tsp dried oregano
- [ ] ¼ cup grated Parmesan cheese

Ingredients for the casserole

- [ ] 2 cups keto marinara
- [ ] 1½ cups whole milk mozzarella cheese, shredded
- [ ] 1 cup whole milk ricotta cheese

Directions for the meatballs

1. Combine all of the meatball ingredients in a medium bowl and mix thoroughly
2. Form into 1.5" meatballs.

3. Place the meatballs on a parchment lined baking sheet, and bake at 375 degrees F. for 15 minutes.

Directions for the casserole

1. Place the meatballs in a casserole dish (13x9) in a single layer.

2. Pour half of the keto marinara sauce over the meatballs.

3. Drop the ricotta cheese evenly over the casserole.

4. Pour the second half of the marinara sauce over the top.

5. Sprinkle the mozzarella cheese over the entire surface.

6. Bake for about 30 minutes at 375 degrees (F).

7. Remove from the oven and let it cool for about five minutes before serving.

Bacon Cheeseburger Pie

Ingredients

1lb. ground beef

2 tsp. onion powder

1 tbsp. dry mined onion

2 whole eggs

1/2 cup mayo

1/4 cup heavy cream

8 oz. shredded cheddar cheese

4 slices bacon

Directions

1. Brown ground beef on medium low heat, with 1tsp. onion powder and 1tbs.p minced onion.
2. Drain fat, season to taste with salt and pepper.
3. Place meat in greased 10" pie plate.
4. Cook bacon to taste then mince into dime-sized portions.
5. Stir 4oz. shredded cheese with bacon and ground beef.
6. Top with 4oz. shredded cheese.
7. Whisk mayo, eggs and cream with a dash of pepper.
8. Pour evenly over meat.
9. Bake at 350F for 30-35 minutes.
10. Let stand for 10 minutes before serving.

Stuffed Jalapeno Peppers

Ingredients

12 medium fresh jalapeno peppers

4 oz. cream cheese, softened

1 1/2 cup (6 oz.) shredded Cheddar or gauda cheese

2-3 slices bacon, cooked and crumbled

Jalapeno pepper sauce

Directions

1. Cut peppers in half lengthwise.
2. Remove seeds membranes.
3. Cook peppers in boiling water 5 to 10 minutes.
4. Drain well.
5. Combine cheeses with bacon and heap into pepper halves and sprinkle with a couple drops of jalapeno pepper sauce.
6. Place on baking sheet and bake in 400F oven for 5 minutes until cheese melts.

Low-carb pizza crust

Ingredients

1 8 oz. package of cream cheese, room temperature

2 eggs

1/4 tsp. ground black pepper

1 tsp garlic powder

1/4 cup grated parmesan cheese

Directions

1. Preheat oven to 375 F.
2. Lightly spray a 9×13 pan with cooking spray.
3. With a handheld mixer, mix cream cheese, eggs, pepper, garlic powder and parmesan cheese until combined.
4. Spread into baking dish (a pan with a lip).
5. Bake for 15-20 minutes, or until golden brown.
6. Let the crust to cool for 10 minutes.
7. Top with low-carb pizza sauce and toppings.
8. Bake 12-15 minutes, until cheese is melted.
9. You can top with pepperoni, onions, mushrooms, and cilantro.

Cheese Mushroom Melt

Ingredients

1 tablespoon olive oil

1/2 tsp garlic, minced

1 large flat mushroom, stalk removed

50g (2oz) Gruyere cheese sliced or another cheese which melts well.

1 tsp. chopped parsley (or 1/2 tsp dried parsley).

Salt and pepper to taste.

Directions

1. Preheat the oven to 220C.
2. Place the mushroom on a baking sheet stalk side up.
3. Season with salt and pepper
4. Mix the oil, garlic and parsley in a small bowl.
5. Brush the mushroom with the oil mixture.
6. Bake in the oven for 5-10 minutes until tender.
7. Remove from oven and add cheese to the well of the mushroom, taking care to leave a small border so your cheese doesn't spill over the sides.
8. Return to the oven and bake for a further 5 minutes

Chapter 7: Dinner Recipes

When the body is in ketosis we are not hungry in general. Some options for dinner can be a healthy meat with steamed, sautéed in coconut oil or raw, non-starchy veggies. To the completed dish I recommend to redound an additional amount of extra virgin olive oil.

Another Great dinner option include soups and stews.

Cauliflower Soup

Ingredients

2 tablespoons olive oil

1 onion, finely chopped

1 cauliflower, broken into pieces

3 cups chicken stock

1 cup cream

Salt and pepper

Directions

1. Preheat oven to 380F.
2. Place onion and cauliflower in a large oven proof dish and drizzle with olive oil.
3. Sprinkle with some salt and pepper.
4. Roast until golden.
5. Place the cauliflower and onions in a large pot and add stock.
6. Bring to a boil.
7. Let it boil 5 minutes, add stock and season with salt and pepper.
8. Pure in a blender and serve with a toasted bred, a little olive oil and some pepper.

Blueberry Almond Muffins

Ingredients

10 gr. Keto-Cal 4:1 Powder

10 gr. frozen blueberries

10 gr. ground almond flour

25 gr. butter

19 gr. eggs, raw, beaten

16 gr. coconut, dried, shredded, unsweetened

1 gr. baking powder

10 gr. (mL) water

Directions

1. Preheat the oven to 350F.
2. Beat the eggs.
3. Mix all the ingredients together.
4. Use a silicone muffin tray or silicone baking cups, as this makes them easier to remove.
5. Cook for 30-35 minutes on 350°F
6. Remove the tray from the oven and allow cooling.

Spinach & Artichoke Soup

Ingredients

4 cups baby spinach leaves

2 cups canned artichoke hearts, drained

1 Tbsp. butter

2 slices provolone cheese

2 oz. Dubliner or cheddar cheese

½ small onion, roughly chopped

2 Tbsp. sour cream

2 cups water

1 tsp. Sriracha hot sauce

½ c heavy cream

½ tsp garlic powder

salt and pepper to taste

Directions

1. Add all ingredients to a blender.
2. Puree.
3. Pour into a medium saucepan and simmer for about 10 - 15 minutes.
4. Taste and adjust seasoning.
5. Add another tablespoon of butter right before serving.

Chicken Soup

Ingredients

3/4 kilo meat for soup

1 lb Chicken breasts

1 tsp. Basil

1 cup Celery

1/2 cup Green beans

1 cup Onions

1 cup Yellow squash

2 cups Zucchini

4 cups Chicken broth

1 tsp. Black pepper

1 tsp. Celery salt

1 1/2 tsp. Salt

Directions

1. Bring the broth to a boil.
2. Add the meat and cook for 2 hours.
3. Add the vegies, chicken cut into cubes, green beans and spices.
4. Stew for another 1/2 hour.
5. Serve with a strew of fresh chopped parsley or dill.

Tomato Soup

Ingredients

2 Tbsp. olive oil

1 sprig oregano

1 medium red onion finely chopped

Salt to taste

4 cloves sliced garlic

28 oz. tomatoes with their juice (1 can)

½ cup Chicken Stock

¾ cup heavy cream

1 tbsp. sriracha sauce

½ cup blue cheese

Greek yogurt for garnish (optional)

Hot sauce

Directions

1. Heat the olive oil in a 4-quart pot over medium heat.
2. Add the onion and a pinch of salt and stew for 2 minutes.
3. Add the garlic and continue to stew for 2 more minutes.
4. Add the tomatoes, their juice, and the stock and bring to a simmer.
5. Add the cream, sriracha sauce and simmer for 10 to 25 minutes.
6. Pour the soup into a blender, add the blue cheese, and blend until smooth..

7. Strain through a fine-mesh strainer into a clean pot, taste, adjust the seasoning

8. Reheat to serve.

9. When serving top with a dollop of Greek yogurt and some extra hot sauce.(optional)

Chicken, Bacon and Tomato Salad

Ingredients

1 large uncooked chicken breast, cut into 1 inch chunks

2 tsp. Canadian Steak Seasoning (Tone's brand is good)

2 tbsp. butter

5 slices bacon

Small tomato, seeded and cut into small chunks

2 ounces Gouda cheese, shredded

Directions

1. Cook the chicken and bacon and put them aside to cool.
2. Sprinkle the chicken with the Canadian Steak seasoning, then sauté it in butter over medium heat until cooked through.
3. Set aside to cool.
4. Cut the bacon strips crosswise into thin strips, and sauté over medium high heat until crispy.
5. Pour off excess grease then drain the bacon on paper towels until cool.

Dressing ingredients

Ingredients

2 tablespoons butter

raw, organic egg yolk, preferably from pastured chickens (makes for richer, tastier yolk)

2 ounces mayonnaise

2 teaspoons lemon juice

1/2 teaspoon salt

Directions

1. Place butter in small sauce pan, and melt over low heat.
2. Do not let it get hot.
3. Remove the melted butter from heat and let cool until warm, but not hot.
4. Add the egg yolk and whisk until the mixture is smooth and glossy.
5. Add the mayonnaise, lemon juice and salt and whisk until smooth.
6. Combine the salad ingredients and the dressing and mix well.
7. Make the dressing a day before serving the salad, and let the flavours meld over night.

Low Carb Bacon Avocado Salad

Ingredients

2 cups fresh, mixed greens

3 slices fried bacon cut in bite size pieces

1 tbsp. sugar free mayonnaise

1 slice of beefsteak tomato, chopped

1/4 avocado, chopped

1-2 tbsp. shredded parmesan or blue cheese.

Directions

1. Cook bacon.
2. Place fresh greens in a salad bowl.
3. Top with 1 tbsp. mayonnaise, chopped avocado and tomato.
4. Place hot bacon on top.
5. Sprinkle shredded cheese on top.

Egg Salad

Ingredients

8 eggs

1/2 cup egg fast coconut oil mayonnaise

1 tsp. ground mustard

Salt & pepper to taste

Directions

1. Slice eggs and then mix in mayonnaise and mustard until well combined.
2. Season with salt & pepper to taste.

Chef Salad

Ingredients

4 large eggs hard-boiled and halved

1 head lettuce or red leaf lettuce

1/2 pound boneless and skinless chicken breast, or ham, grilled and diced

2 bacon slices, cooked and crumbled

1/2 cup cherry tomatoes, halved

4 medium onions, sliced thin

2 medium celery stalks, diced

1 Medium avocado, diced

4 teaspoons favourite salad dressing

Direction

1. Hard-boil eggs, cool and remove shells.
2. Cook bacon and crumble, grill chicken or ham and dice.
3. Wash and chop vegetables.
4. Divide lettuce between plates, top with vegetables, eggs, avocado and meats.
5. Top with Salad Dressing.

Shrimps Salad

Ingredients

2 14-ounce bags frozen, cooked salad shrimp, thawed

4 stalks celery, thinly sliced

1/2 small onion, finely minced

4 small tomatoes

1 1/2 cups mayonnaise

3 tsp. lemon juice

1/4 tsp. Old Bay Seafood Seasoning

salt and pepper to taste

8 cups mixed salad greens

4 tbsp. chopped green onions

Directions

1. Defrost the shrimp it in a colander and running cold water over it.
2. Set aside to drain thoroughly.
3. Slice the celery and mince the onion.
4. In a small mixing bowl, combine the mayonnaise, lemon juice, Old Bay Seafood Seasoning, salt, and pepper.
5. Whisk to combine.
6. Put the defrosted shrimp, sliced celery, and minced onion in a large bowl and toss to combine them.
7. Pour the mayonnaise mixture over the top and gently toss to evenly distribute the dressing.

8. Cover the shrimp salad tightly with plastic wrap.

9. Refrigerate the salad mixture for at least one hour (but no more than 24 hours).

10. Slice each of the tomatoes into eight wedges just before serving.

11. Remove the tomatoes cores and the seeds.

12. Put the tomato wedges on paper towels to drain for a few minutes.

13. Slice the cucumber into thin slices.

14. Chop the green onions.

15. Distribute the salad greens on dinner plates.

16. Mound the shrimp salad mixture in the centre of the greens.

17. Arrange the tomato wedges and cucumber slices around shrimps.

18. Sprinkle 1 tablespoon of the chopped green onions on top of salad.

Chapter 8: Keto Desserts

Here are some great options for amazing ketogenic desserts, for those of you who have a sweet tooth. You can eat sweets and still rep the full benefits from this keto diet.

Chocolate dessert

Ingredients

100g (4 oz.) dark (semisweet) chocolate

50g (2 oz.) unsalted butter, plus some for preparing the dishes

2 eggs

2 tablespoons light sugar

2 tablespoons flour

½ teaspoon vanilla extract

pinch of salt

Directions

1. Set your oven to 200°C (400°F) and grease 2 small ovenproof dishes with butter.
2. Place them on a baking tray.
3. Chop the chocolate and place in a microwaveable dish.
4. Add the butter and microwave in 30-second bursts until melted.
5. In a medium bowl, beat the eggs and sugar together with the salt and vanilla until very well combined..

6. Stir in the slightly cooled chocolate, then mix in the flour until just combined. Don't over-beat.

7. Divide the mixture between the dishes and cook for 12 minutes or until the top is just beginning to crack and then remove from the oven.

8. Let them sit for 5 minutes before serving.

9. A delicious variation is to serve them with cream or vanilla ice cream.

Chocolate Coconut Keto Ice Cream

Ingredients

1/2 cup of full fat coconut milk

1 tbsp. of unsweetened cocoa or cacao powder

1 tbsp. of organic heavy whipping cream

Directions

1. Whip the cream for 2 minutes and place it in the freezer for 20-30 minutes (if more it will be frozen, if less it will be like pudding).
2. You could add a tablespoon of some stevia (optional)

Chocolate Ice Cream

Ingredients

2 large Egg Yolks

3 cups Heavy Cream

4 large Eggs (Whole)

3/4 cup Cocoa Powder (Unsweetened)

3/4 cup Sucralose Based Sweetener (Sugar Substitute)

1/4 tsp Salt

2 tsps. Vanilla Extract

1/2 tsp Pure Almond Extract

Directions

1. Pour heavy cream into a heavy-bottomed 3-quart saucepan and place over medium heat.
2. Allow to simmer but do not boil. Remove from heat and set aside.
3. In a large mixing bowl, combine the eggs, yolks, cocoa powder, sugar substitute and salt.
4. With an electric mixer on medium, beat until thickened and smooth, 2 to 3 minutes, scraping sides of bowl with a rubber spatula.
5. Using a ladle, remove about a cup of the hot cream from the pan, and gradually whisk into egg mixture (this tempers the eggs so they won't curdle).
6. While whisking, pour tempered egg mixture into remaining cream in saucepan.

7. Place over medium heat and whisk until slightly thickened and coats the back of a wooden spoon; temperature should not go over 170°F.

8. Pour into a clean bowl, whisk in extracts and let stand until custard is cooled to room temperature, about 1 1/2 hours.

9. Refrigerate 2 hours, until well chilled, or cover with plastic wrap and refrigerate overnight for more flavour.

10. Freeze in ice cream maker according to manufacturer's directions.

11. Serve immediately for soft serve ice cream.

12. For firm ice cream, place in an airtight container and freeze 2 to 4 hours or overnight.

Ketogenic Cheesecake

Ingredients

8oz cream cheese

4oz heavy cream

4T sour cream

4T Sugar free syrup or vanilla extract + sweetener to taste

Directions

Blend all ingredients in the mixer and whip until it forms stiff peaks.

Cheese Cupcakes

Ingredients

1/2 stick of butter

1/2 cup almond flour

2 8 oz. packages of soft cream cheese

3/4 cup of Splenda

1 tsp vanilla

2 eggs

Directions

1. Pre-heat oven to 350 degrees.
2. Melt the butter for the crust and stir in the almond flour, until the desired consistency.
3. Place a small amount in the bottom of a cupcake liner and pat down to form the crust.
4. Add the cream cheese, eggs, Splenda, and vanilla to the bowl and mix on medium speed until the mixture is smooth.
5. When the filling smooth, fill the cupcake liners almost to the top.
6. Bake in the oven for 15-17 minutes.
7. Cool first, and then chill overnight.

Coffee Ricotta Mousse

Ingredients

2 1/2 teaspoons dry gelatine

1/2 cup hot brewed coffee

2 cups Ricotta cheese

1 tsp. instant espresso

1 tsp. vanilla extract

1 tsp. vanilla liquid stevia

pinch salt

1 cup heavy whipping cream

shaved sugar free chocolate to garnish

Directions

1. Pour the gelatine into the hot coffee and stir until dissolved.
2. Set aside to cool slightly.
3. Add the ricotta, espresso, vanilla extract, stevia and salt to a mixer.
4. Blend until well combined.
5. Pour in cooled coffee gelatine mixture and blend until smooth.
6. Pour in whipping cream and blend on high until thickened and whipped.
7. Spoon into serving dishes and garnish with shaved chocolate.
8. Place in refrigerator for 2 hours.

Sweet Balls

Ingredients

2 tbsp. of sweetener

2 tbsp. of water

2 cups of almond flour

1 tbsp. almond extract

1 tbsp. of vanilla extract

Ingredients For Toppings

Coconut Flakes

Sesame

Cinnamon

Cocoa Powder

Directions

1. Mix the 2 tbsp. of sweetener with the 2 tbsp. of water.
2. Add the almond extract and the vanilla extract.
3. Add the 2 cups of almond flour.
4. Mix them well.
5. Form little balls.
6. Roll them in the toppings you prefer (coconut, cacao, chocolate, hemp hearts, chia seeds)
7. Place them in the fridge for 1 hr.

Eggnog Pie

Ingredients

4 large eggs

8 tbsp. unsalted butter, melted

1/8 tsp. kosher salt

1 tbsp. vanilla extract

1/4 tsp. baking powder

3/4 cup unsweetened coconut flakes

2 tbsp. Mile High Biscuit Mix

2 tbsp. coconut flour

1/2 cups heavy cream

1/3 cup water

1/8 cup sugar free vanilla syrup

1/4 cup dark rum—or 1 teaspoon Cook's Pure Rum Extract

1/3 cup Granular Swerve, measure before powdering

8-10 drops concentrated vanilla stevia drops, to taste

1/2 tsp. nutmeg, freshly grated if possible

1/2 tsp. ground cinnamon

Directions

1. Preheat oven to 325°.
2. Spray 9 to 10-inch pie pan with coconut oil cooking spray.
3. Place all ingredients in a blender and blend until smooth.

4. Pour into previously prepared 9 to 10-inch pie pan.

5. Place pie pan on a baking sheet pan with sides.

6. Place on the middle rack.

7. Pour warm water about half way up into the outer baking pan.

8. Bake in a preheated 325° oven for about 45-50 minutes.

9. The centre should jiggle slightly but toothpick inserted into the centre should come away clean.

10. Tent it with aluminium foil at about the 25 minute to avoid over-browning.

11. Cool completely on a wire rack then cover and refrigerate a minimum of 4 hours or preferably overnight.

12. The pie tastes better the next day.

French Pie

For Walnut Pie Crust

½ cup walnuts

1 cup Almond Flour

⅓ cup Ground Flax Seed

⅓ cup Protein Powder

2 tbsp. Gentle Sweet

⅛ tsp. salt

⅓ cup (6 tablespoons) ghee, or butter, melted

French Pie Filling

6 Ounces (1½ Sticks) Salted Butter, Soft

1¼ Cups Gentle Sweet

¼ Cup Heavy Cream

3½ Ounces Unsweetened Baking Chocolate Squares, Melted

4 Large Pasteurized Eggs

2 Tsp Vanilla Extract

½ Tsp. Stevia Or Gentle Sweet

¾ Cup Heavy Cream

Chocolate Shavings From 2 Squares Of Chocolate

Directions

1. Preheat oven to 350 degrees.

2. Make the Walnut Pie Crust: spray a pie plate with baking spray.

3. Put the walnuts in a food processor and process them until finely ground, (but not walnut butter!).

4. In a medium bowl, add all of the dry ingredients and stir together, thoroughly.

5. Melt the butter or ghee and add to the dry ingredients stirring together. The mixture should clump up easily and hold its shape when squeezed firmly. If not, add a little bit more oil.

6. Add walnut crust ingredients to the pie plate and begin to press it firmly into the sides and bottom of the plate.

7. With the tines of a fork, poke holes on the bottom and sides of the crust so it doesn't puff up in the oven.

8. Bake the crust for 10 minutes, or until it begins to turn a nice golden brown.

9. Let cool completely.

Directions for the French Pie

1. Finely chop the unsweetened baking chocolate and put in a microwaveable bowl.

2. Heat on high 30 seconds at a time until almost melted. The residual heat from the bowl should take care of melting the rest.

3. Put the butter and the sweetener in a stand mixer or in a large mixing bowl.

4. Fit the paddle attachment onto the mixer and beat the butter and sweetener on medium speed for about 2 minutes. Scrape the bowl.

5. Add the melted chocolate and mix for 1 minute. Scrape down the bowl thoroughly.

6. Add ¼ cup of heavy cream, vanilla and stevia, beating for 2 minutes more. Remove the paddle attachment, and scrape the filling back into the bowl.

7. Add the whisk attachment and turn the stand mixer back on medium speed.

8. Add one egg and let the mixer run for about 5 minutes. Scrape the bowl. Add another egg and again let the machine run for about 5 minutes. Follow this procedure with each egg, making sure to scrape the bowl after each addition.

9. Finish mixing with a quick burst at high speed and spread the filling into the pie shell and refrigerate.

10. Whip the ¾ cup of heavy cream with sweetener and top the pie.

Lemon Pie

Ingredients

1 Basic Almond Pie Crust (recipe below)

¾ cup lemon juice

½ cup sweetener of your choice

tbsp. corn-starch

4 large eggs

4 large egg yolks

Lemon zest from the lemons used

6 tbsp. salted butter, cut into pieces

½ tsp. sweetener

1 cup heavy cream or coconut cream

⅛ tsp. xanthan gum (as stabilizer)

½ cup heavy cream or coconut cream

3 tbsp. additional sweetener

Directions

1. Make the lemon curd the day before or in the morning so that it has time to chill.

2. Prepare the Basic Almond Pie Crust according to instructions and let cool.

3. Lemon Curd: Measure the sweetener and corn-starch and put them in a medium pot. Stir together.

4. Roll the lemons on the counter to get them juicy, then zest the lemons adding the zest to the sweetener.

5. Separate 4 eggs and add the yolks to the sweetener in the pot.

6. Add the 4 whole eggs to the pot and whisk the eggs and sweetener together.

7. Juice the lemons and measure ¾ cup. Strain the lemon juice and stir it into the eggs.

8. Turn the heat to medium and continuously whisk the mixture until it begins to thicken.

9. Turn the heat down to medium-low and continue whisking. The lemon curd will thicken immediately.

10. Remove the pot from the heat and continue to stir with the whisk for one minute more.

11. Pour into a clean container and add more sweetener and salted butter incorporating completely.

12. To cool, place a piece of plastic wrap right on top of the low carb lemon curd and refrigerate.

To Assemble the Low Carb Lemon Pie

1. Whip 1 cup of the heavy cream with about ⅔ of the sweetener and the xanthan gum until the whipped cream is very stiff.

2. Stir ⅓ of the whipped cream into the lemon curd to lighten it.

3. Fold ½ of the remaining whipped cream into the lemon curd and finally fold in the rest.

4. Scrape the pie filling into the pie crust and smooth out to the edges

5. Whip the remaining whipped cream with the remaining sweetener until stiff.

6. Stir to soften and break-up the whipped cream just a bit.

7. Spread over the filling and refrigerate at least four hours to over-night.

How to make the Almond Pie Crust

Ingredients

1 ½ cups (135 grams) Almond Flour

⅓ cup ground G Flax Seed

⅓ cup vanilla whey protein powder (or egg white protein powder)

6 tbs. salted butter, melted

2 tbs. sweetener

¼ tsp salt

Directions

1. Preheat oven to 350. Measure the sweetener.
2. Measure all of the dry ingredients into a smallish bowl, add the sweetener and mix together.
3. Melt the butter, (or olive oil) and pour over the crust ingredients.
4. Mix with a fork or a rubber spatula until the butter is incorporated and the mixture clumps.
5. Press firmly into an oven -proof pie plate. Dock all over with a fork.
6. Bake 10 minutes until golden and set.
7. Cool before eating.

Banana Cream Pie

Ingredients

1 batch Low Carb Walnut Pie Crust as per directions in the previous recipes

Banana Cream Filling

1 cup heavy cream

⅓ cup almond milk

⅓ cup sweetener

2 tablespoons corn starch (or arrowroot)

⅛ tsp. xanthan gum

3 large egg yolk

2 large eggs

1 tsp. vanilla

1 tsp. banana extract

pinch salt

2 tbsp. butter

½ tsp stevia

For Filling and Topping

1½ cups heavy cream

sweetener to taste

Directions

Make the Low Carb Walnut Pie Crust as per instructions Cool completely.

Banana Cream Filling

1. Ready a strainer by the stove. Place the cream and almond milk in a medium sauce pan, and turn the heat to medium - low.

2. Add the sweetener, corn starch, xanthan gum and salt to a medium heat-proof mixing bowl and mix together with a small whisk.

3. Separate 3 of the eggs adding the yolks to the dry ingredients in the bowl.

4. Add the two whole eggs to the bowl and whisk together.

5. If bubbling and simmering hasn't occurred around the sides of the saucepan, turn the heat up to medium until it does.

6. Turn-off the heat and while whisking the egg mixture continuously, pour all of the cream into the mixing bowl in a thin stream.

7. Put the pot back on the stove and scrape the egg and cream mixture into the pot. Quickly rinse out the bowl, swipe with a paper towel, and set next to the stove with the strainer over the top.

8. Turn the heat to medium low and begin whisking the pastry cream. After about 2½ minutes it will start to thicken-up slightly. Whisk a little faster. At about the 3 - 3½ minute mark, it will begin to thicken. Whisk briskly and cook for 1 minute more but don't let the mixture boil or the eggs will scramble.

9. Turn off the heat and remove the pot from the stove.

10. Still whisking briskly for another minute.

11. Whisk in the vanilla, banana extract, stevia and butter.

12. Then, pour the pastry cream through the strainer, catching any cooked egg bits.

13. To cool, push a piece of plastic wrap right on top of the surface of the pastry cream and place in the refrigerator.

14. Whip the cream until firm but not totally stiff. Sweeten to taste.

15. Remove the banana cream filling from the refrigerator and beat it with a hand mixer until it is lightened a little - just 30 seconds or so.

16. Add ¼ of the whipped cream to the filling and fold it in with a rubber spatula.

17. Add another ¼ of the whipped cream, again folding it into the filling.

18. Put the filling into the crust and smooth to the edges.

19. Add the remaining whipped cream to the top and spread over the banana cream filling.

20. Refrigerate several hours before serving.

Conclusion

Researchers highlighted some of the areas of active research in this field and they found the ketogenic diet efficacious and relatively saf,e with impressive results.. This is a promising nutritional approach of low-carb style of eating which means carbohydrate restriction.

Using the remarkable ability of humans to adapt to existence conditions, the removal of high-glycaemic carbohydrates such as sugar and flour from the diets of diabetics was found to be a successful method of controlling hyperglycaemia.

Dr Atkins, an American physician, discovered the way in which a diet low in carbohydrates can help the body burn fat instead of glucose, to create energy.

The diet seems to be an effective way of losing weight that suits many people.

However, eating a low-carbohydrate and high-protein diet has different effects on different systems in the body and certainly in different people. These are not fully understood; therefore check with your doctor before starting any nutritional protocol, and especially if you have kidney problems.

I would not advise you ketogenic diet if you are a type 1 diabetic.

www.ingramcontent.com/pod-product-compliance
Lightning Source LLC
Chambersburg PA
CBHW072013290526

45787CB00013B/890